THE SPARKS THAT ENDURE

COMPANION WORKBOOK

A Reflective Workbook for Recovery, Meaning, and Connection

BY CLOVIS RAYMOND, MD

Designed for individuals, families, peers, and clinicians

Copyright © 2025 by Clovis Raymond, MD

All rights reserved. No part of this publication may be reproduced, stored in a retrieval system, or transmitted in any form or by any means—electronic, mechanical, photocopying, recording, or otherwise—without the prior written permission from **the author**, except in the case of brief quotations embodied in critical articles or reviews.

ISBN: Workbook: 979-8-9935477-2-5

Library of Congress Control Number: Pending

Cataloging-in-Publication Data: Pending

Publication year: 2025

Edited by Cynthia Constantino
Cover and interior design by Andy Magee

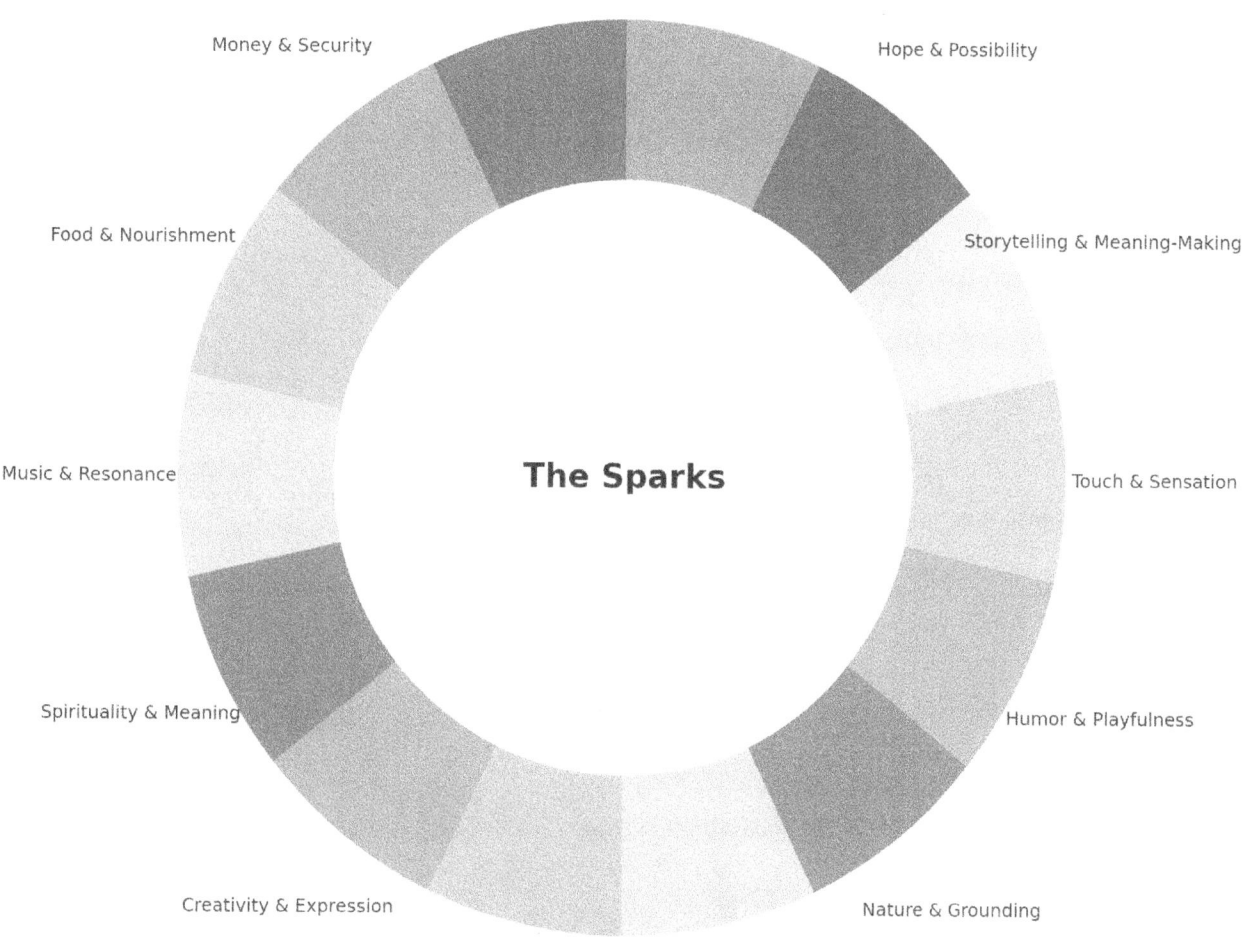

Contents

Dedication 6
Welcome Letter 7
How to Use This Workbook 9
Module 1 11
Module 2 13
Module 3 15
Module 4 17
Module 5 19
Module 6 21
Module 7 23
Module 8 25
Module 9 27
Module 10 29
Module 11 31
Module 12 33
Module 13 35
Module 14 37
Module 15 39
Spark Self-Assessment Tool (General) 39
Clinician Sparks Assessment Tool 45
The Spark Wheel 81
Module 16 85
References 87

Praise for The Sparks That Endure

"In The Sparks That Endure, Dr. Clovis Raymond illuminates the often-overlooked truth that core human drives—such as the need for meaning, intimacy, and self-expression—do not disappear in the face of serious mental illness. With clinical insight and deep compassion, he challenges us to see our patients not solely through the lens of pathology, but through the light of their enduring humanity. This book is a necessary addition to the evolving field of person-centered psychiatry."

—Mardoche Sidor, MD, Quadruple Board-Certified Psychiatrist, Founder of SWEET Institute, Author of Mindset, Mood & Memory

"Dr. Raymond, in his book, The Sparks That Endure, brilliantly, elegantly, and humanistically demonstrates how one is more than their illness. This holistic point of view mirrors what I have witnessed for years in my therapy room. Dr. Raymond refreshingly highlights the common human needs of connection, meaning, and purpose—the 'sparks' that refuse to be extinguished despite a debilitating illness and its significance in establishing therapeutic rapport and providing treatment. This book is a must-read and I'll be recommending it highly to every clinician and non-clinician alike."

—Dr. Andreia Harris, PhD, Licensed Clinical Psychologist; Clinical Supervisor at Health & Hospitals Corporation (Rikers Island); Former Deputy Director of Mental Health at Rikers Island; Former Training Director in Psychology at Mount Sinai Hospital/Elmhurst Hospital Center; Former Executive Clinical Director at On-Site Psychological Services; Former Director of Psychotic Disorders Program at NY Hospital, Cornell/Westchester

"In both medicine and nursing education, we're taught to assess symptoms, manage conditions, and measure outcomes. But rarely are we trained to see the enduring desires—the sparks—that remain alive beneath a diagnosis. In The Sparks That Endure, Dr. Clovis Raymond delivers a powerful, paradigm-shifting message: that even amid serious mental illness, individuals hold onto deep and vital longings—connection, joy, purpose, creativity. As a physician and the director of a nursing institute, I see this book as essential reading for clinicians, educators, and caregivers alike. It challenges us to treat not just the illness, but the humanity that persists within it."

—Roger Fimerlus, MD, Founder & Director, Hearts Institute Nursing School, Florida

"In a world where wellness is often reduced to quick fixes and surface solutions, The Sparks That Endure *dares to go deeper. Dr. Clovis Raymond brings compassion, clarity, and hard-earned wisdom to the conversation around mental health, reminding us that healing is not about erasing struggle but reconnecting to the drives that make us feel alive. Dr. Clovis Raymond doesn't just talk about mental illness—he listens deeply to what still burns beneath it. As a radio host who hears real stories every day, I can tell you this: people want to be seen, not just diagnosed. This book does exactly that. It's powerful, human, and long overdue."*

—Seema Roc, Director of Community Affairs; Radio Host

"In The Sparks That Endure, *Dr. Clovis Raymond brings a wealth of insight as a professor, psychiatrist, scholar, and practitioner. His perspective is global, cross-cultural, and combines scholarly research with profound practicality."*

—Dr. F. Adam Souffrant, Lead Pastor, Maranatha Evangelical Church of the

Nazarene, Philadelphia, PA; Church Consultant; Member at Large, New York State Association of Protestant Chaplains

"As someone who has guided countless young people through life's pivotal transitions—from high school to higher education, from confusion to clarity—I find The Sparks That Endure *to be a profound and necessary work. Dr. Clovis Raymond has captured something we often miss in both education and mental health: that the core human longings—like meaning, connection, creativity, and joy—do not disappear in illness. They persist. They endure. They guide. Whether in my role as a school counselor, a Sunday school director, or a Christian mentor, I've seen firsthand how these sparks sustain hope and ignite transformation, even in the most discouraged hearts. This book is not only a compassionate guide for professionals—it's a mirror for every one of us who believes healing is not just possible, but purposeful."*

—Denet Alexandre, MA, School Guidance Counselor; Director of Christian

Education; Chair, Board of Trustees, Falkenstein Library; Christian Ministry Counselor, Spring Valley, NY

"I appreciate Dr. Raymond's adroitness in peeling the nuances which envelop the indestructible sparks that feed the intricate webs of our humanity, even when affected by the most severe forms of mental disorders. Through his sympathetic therapeutic alliance with his patients, he has uncovered their enduring determination to thrive and to generate hope. This book is an indispensable tool for mental health practitioners, researchers, scholars, and anyone who is concerned with mental health recovery."

—Dr. Emmanuel Charles, LMSW, Former Forensic Program Administrator and Forensic Treatment Team Leader (Kirby Forensic Psychiatric Center)

Dedication

For every patient, peer, and caregiver who never stopped looking for meaning—even in the darkest times. This workbook is for you, and for the sparks that refused to go out.

Welcome Letter

Dear Reader,

Welcome to the companion workbook for The Sparks That Endure. This resource is for anyone navigating serious mental illness—whether you're living with it, supporting someone who is, or working in a professional role. Each section is based on a core human drive, what we call a spark.

If you've picked up this workbook, I already know something about you: you believe that healing is possible. You believe that people are more than their symptoms, more than their diagnosis. You believe in something deeper, spark that endures.

This workbook is a companion to my book, *The Sparks That Endure*. It's not a textbook. It's not a checklist. It's a space—for reflection, discovery, and truth-telling. Whether you're living with mental illness, supporting someone who is, or working in the field of care, you're welcome here. Your experience is valid. Your perspective matters.

The Sparks That Endure: Companion Workbook is more than a collection of exercises—it's a map back to what makes life worth living.

Designed for individuals, clinicians, families, and recovery groups, this workbook invites reflection on the enduring human drives—sex, food, music, meaning, creativity, and more—that persist even through serious mental illness.

Throughout these pages, you'll find questions, tools, and stories meant to help you connect to the things that bring you joy, meaning, and energy, the sparks that keep us going even when everything else feels dim.

So take your time. Write in the margins. Circle, highlight, or draw. Use what speaks to you. Skip what doesn't. This is your journey.

With compassion, structure, and insight, psychiatrist Clovis Raymond, MD offers readers a way to reconnect with sparks that never fully go out.

Use this workbook to reflect, journal, assess, and grow. The goal is not to complete it quickly, but to engage with it honestly. Your spark is waiting.

With gratitude,
Clovis Raymond, MD

How to Use This Workbook

This workbook was designed to meet you where you are. It includes stories, reflection prompts, journaling pages, spark check-ins, and tools for both personal and clinical use. Here's how you might use it:

- Read a Spark chapter in the book, then complete the matching section here.
- Use the Self-Assessment Tool to reflect on which Sparks are active—and which are dimmed.
- Fill out the Spark Journal pages after a therapy session, support group, or personal insight.
- As a clinician, use the Clinician Spark Toolkit to integrate strengths and meaning into care plans.

There is no wrong way to use this workbook. It's yours.

Make it messy. Make it honest. Let it reflect who you are and where you're going.

What Are Sparks?

Sparks are core human drives—like love, music, food, and freedom—that ignite our sense of purpose and identity. Even in the depths of illness, these sparks often survive. This workbook helps uncover, explore, and nurture them.

Spark Self-Inventory

Rate each spark below from 0 (not present) to 5 (very strong in my life):

- Sex and Connection: _____
- Money and Autonomy: _____
- Food and Nourishment: _____
- Music and Rhythm: _____
- Spirituality and Meaning: _____
- Creativity and Expression: _____
- Movement and Agency: _____
- Rituals and Continuity: _____
- Nature and Grounding: _____
- Humor and Lightness: _____
- Hope: _____
- Touch: _____
- Storytelling: _____
- Freedom: _____

Guided Spark Mapping Exercise

On a blank sheet of paper or the space below, draw your 'spark map'. Place yourself in the center and surround yourself with the sparks that feel most alive to you today. Use lines, colors, or symbols to show which are connected or most important. Reflect on how these sparks have changed over time.

Module 1

Sex and Intimacy: The Spark of Connection and Desire

Sex and intimacy are often left out of the conversation in mental health, yet they remain some of the most enduring sources of vitality and connection. For many people—whether navigating symptoms, medications, stigma, or past trauma—the experience of closeness, touch, desire, and partnership still matters deeply.

This module isn't about performance or expectations. It's about honoring your relationship to intimacy—whatever form that takes. It's about remembering that you are worthy of touch, love, and belonging.

'Even when I was at my worst,' one patient shared, 'I still wanted to be held.' That statement has stayed with me. Because so many people, even at their most vulnerable, still carry a longing to connect.

Reflection Prompts

- When do I feel most connected to others?
- What role does touch or affection play in my life?
- Have medications or symptoms impacted my sexuality or relationships?
- What kind of intimacy do I long for (emotional, physical, spiritual)?
- What are my boundaries, and how do I communicate them?

Spark Journal

Use this space to write freely about your experiences with sex, intimacy, and connection. No judgment. Just honesty.

_____

_____

_____

_____

_____

_____

Try This: Rekindle the Spark

Choose one small action that supports intimacy in your life this week. That might mean initiating a meaningful conversation, setting a boundary, practicing self-touch with care, or expressing desire. Intimacy is not just about others—it's about how you relate to your own body and needs.

Clinician Insight

In clinical settings, conversations about sex are often avoided. But honoring the sexual and relational health of patients can enhance trust and therapeutic alliance. Consider asking: 'What brings you joy or closeness?' rather than just focusing on risk. Normalize these discussions across diagnoses and demographics.

Module 2

Money and Security: The Spark of Safety and Survival

Money is more than math. It's survival, dignity, independence, and sometimes even shame. For people living with serious mental illness, money can become a source of both stress and motivation—a symbol of autonomy or a daily reminder of struggle.

One man once told me: 'Even when I had nothing, I still dreamed about winning the lottery. Not to buy things—but to feel safe.' That dream, that desire for stability, lives in many of us.

This module invites you to think about your relationship with money—not just as currency, but as a spark. What does security mean to you? Where do you feel empowered, and where do you feel stuck?

Reflection Prompts

- When have I felt financially safe or unsafe?
- What emotions come up when I think about money?
- How has mental illness affected my finances (or vice versa)?
- Do I feel in control of my financial life?
- What would financial freedom look like for me?

Spark Journal

Write about your experiences with money—past, present, or imagined. You might explore budgeting, spending, receiving help, or planning for your future.

_____

_____

_____

_____

_____

_____

_____

Try This: Make a Micro-Plan

Choose one small money-related action this week that supports your wellbeing. This could be tracking spending for a day, calling about a benefit you're eligible for, or simply listing your financial goals. Money sparks grow in small steps.

Clinician Insight

Money often intersects with psychiatric care—through disability benefits, housing, medication costs, or delusions. Rather than avoiding the topic, clinicians can explore the emotional and symbolic meaning of money in a patient's life. Asking 'What does having enough mean to you?' can open powerful insights.

Module 3

Food and Nourishment: The Spark of Sustenance and Memory

Food is more than fuel. It's culture, comfort, control, and connection. For many people facing mental illness, food can also become complicated—shaped by medication side effects, access issues, eating disorders, or trauma.

Still, food often remains a vivid spark. It ties us to people, to holidays, to smells from childhood. I remember a woman in inpatient care who lit up when we mentioned coconut rice. She hadn't spoken in days, but just that memory pulled her back.

This module is about reclaiming food—not just as a nutritional need, but as a source of grounding, meaning, and pleasure.

Reflection Prompts

- What foods remind me of home or family?
- How do I feel when I eat alone versus with others?
- Have my symptoms or meds affected my appetite or relationship with food?
- What does nourishment mean to me beyond calories?
- Are there rituals around food that I miss or crave?

Spark Journal

Describe your relationship with food. You can explore comfort foods, meals that bring joy, or struggles with nourishment.

___
___
___
___
___
___
___
___

Try This: Savor a Meal

Pick one meal this week to eat slowly and with full attention. Notice the texture, the smell, the memory it might hold. Whether you eat alone or with others, allow this moment to be a spark—not just consumption, but care.

Clinician Insight

Nutrition often intersects with psychiatric treatment through weight changes, appetite shifts, or metabolic concerns. But food is also a spark—anchoring people in routine, culture, and embodiment. Ask about what patients enjoy, not just what they're avoiding. Explore how food practices reflect autonomy, connection, or distress.

Module 4

Music and Resonance: The Spark of Rhythm and Recognition

Music reaches us in ways words sometimes can't. A single melody can spark memory, soothe anxiety, or break through a fog of depression. For people living with mental illness, music often remains accessible—even when language, focus, or motivation fade.

One man I treated told me he couldn't recall the names of his doctors, but he could still hum every verse of a Marvin Gaye song. Music had become his memory anchor, his companion through psychosis and loneliness.

This module honors music not just as entertainment, but as medicine—something that vibrates in the body, reminds us who we are, and connects us to a bigger world.

Reflection Prompts

- What songs have stayed with me during hard times?
- Are there certain rhythms, voices, or instruments that bring me comfort?
- How does music affect my emotions or energy?
- Do I use music to connect, to escape, to regulate?
- What role does music play in my healing journey?

Spark Journal

Write about the songs, lyrics, or sounds that have shaped you. Let this be a playlist of memory, identity, or recovery.

_____
_____
_____
_____
_____
_____
_____
_____

Try This: Make a Spark Playlist

Create a playlist of songs that uplift you, calm you, or speak to your story. Title it 'My Spark Tracks.' Play it during a walk, a shower, or a moment of rest. Let music remind you that you're still here—and still in rhythm.

Clinician Insight

Music can serve as a therapeutic bridge, especially for patients with cognitive impairment, catatonia, or trauma. Ask: 'What music helps you feel like yourself?' or 'Is there a song that's carried you through?' Musical memory often survives even when verbal memory fades.

Module 5

Spirituality and Meaning: The Spark of Faith, Purpose, and Inner Light

Spirituality is not just about religion. It's about searching for meaning, finding connection to something larger, and holding on to hope even in darkness. For people living with serious mental illness, spiritual beliefs can be a source of comfort—or at times, confusion. But even amid psychosis or despair, many individuals speak of a guiding force, a sacred presence, or a sense that their lives still hold purpose.

One woman told me, 'Even when I lost my mind, I didn't lose my soul.' That stayed with me. Because often, meaning endures even when cognition is fractured.

This module honors the spiritual spark—however you define it. Whether through prayer, meditation, music, or quiet reflection, you are invited to reconnect with your deeper sense of meaning.

Reflection Prompts

- What gives my life meaning?
- Do I feel connected to a higher power, nature, ancestors, or community?
- When have I felt spiritually grounded, even during crisis?
- Are there spiritual practices that help me feel safe or whole?
- How have mental illness and spirituality interacted in my life?

Spark Journal

Write about a moment that felt sacred, purposeful, or healing. Or reflect on your spiritual journey—questions, losses, growth.

_____
_____
_____
_____
_____
_____
_____

Try This: Create a Meaning Ritual

Choose a small daily ritual that reconnects you to meaning—lighting a candle, reading a sacred text, sitting in silence, reciting an affirmation, or stepping outside. Let it be a reminder that you are more than your diagnosis—you are still becoming.

Clinician Insight

Spiritual beliefs often influence how patients understand their illness and recovery. Some may interpret symptoms as religious experiences. Others may draw strength from faith. Normalize these conversations. Ask: 'What helps you make sense of this experience?' or 'Are there spiritual practices that support you?' Avoid pathologizing faith, and explore both meaning and distress with curiosity.

Module 6

Creativity and Expression: The Spark of Voice, Imagination, and Inner Truth

Creativity isn't only about painting or poetry. It's about expressing what's inside when words fall short. It's about making meaning, even in the midst of struggle. For people living with mental illness, creativity can be a lifeline—helping to name pain, reclaim identity, or simply offer relief.

I once knew a man who couldn't speak after his first psychotic break. But he began sketching faces—hundreds of them. He told me, 'These are the people in my head.' Art gave him back a voice.

This module is about your creative spark—however it shows up. Whether through drawing, storytelling, journaling, cooking, or dreaming, you have something worth expressing.

Reflection Prompts

- When do I feel most creative or expressive?
- What helped me feel seen or heard in the past?
- What forms of art, music, or movement help me express myself?
- Do I give myself permission to be messy or imperfect in creating?
- How has mental illness influenced my creativity—or vice versa?

Spark Journal

Reflect on a time when you made something from emotion. What did it teach you? What parts of yourself emerged?

_____
_____
_____
_____
_____
_____
_____

Try This: Create Something Small

Choose a simple act of expression—write a short poem, doodle on a napkin, build a playlist that tells your story. Let go of perfection. Just create. This is about freedom, not mastery.

Clinician Insight

Creative expression often opens emotional doors that verbal therapy cannot. For many patients, art, journaling, and music offer safer paths into trauma, identity, or joy. Encourage creative exploration in recovery planning. Ask: 'Is there a way you express what you're going through—even if it's not in words?'

Module 7

Movement and Embodiment: The Spark of Motion, Presence, and Reconnection

The body holds so much—stress, memory, trauma, vitality. For those living with serious mental illness, the connection to the body can sometimes feel disrupted. Movement can become stiff from medication, disembodied from dissociation, or weighed down by depression.

But the body also offers a path back. Gentle motion, stretching, walking, or dancing can ground a person when their mind feels chaotic. I once saw a patient begin to heal through yoga after years of silence. He said, 'My body remembered what my mouth couldn't say.'

This module explores how reconnecting with your body—through movement, breath, and stillness—can be a form of healing, expression, and spark.

Reflection Prompts

- How do I feel in my body today?
- What types of movement make me feel more alive, free, or grounded?
- Have I ever used movement (walking, dancing, stretching) to cope with strong feelings?
- Are there parts of my body or movement history that carry shame, pride, or pain?
- How does my mental health affect how I move or inhabit my body?

Spark Journal

Write about your relationship with movement. What does your body remember? What kind of motion feels like home?

_____

_____

_____

_____

_____

_____

_____

_____

Try This: Mindful Movement

Take five minutes to move intentionally—walk outside, stretch slowly, or sway to music. Focus on your breath, your posture, your rhythm. Let movement be a form of self-connection, not performance.

Clinician Insight

Movement-based therapies can reintroduce embodiment in ways that traditional talk therapy cannot. Patients with trauma histories, catatonia, or mood disorders may benefit from body-oriented practices like dance therapy, yoga, or walking groups. Consider asking: 'What kind of movement helps you feel most like yourself?'

Module 8

Rituals and Structure: The Spark of Safety, Rhythm, and Identity

Rituals are more than habits. They are moments of rhythm, intention, and meaning. They help us feel safe in a world that can be chaotic. For individuals living with serious mental illness, rituals can offer stability—whether it's the morning coffee, a bedtime prayer, or checking the same lock three times.

Sometimes, rituals can become rigid or distressing. But often, they're a form of grounding, a way to make sense of time, space, and self. One patient told me, 'If I light a candle every evening, I feel like the day had shape. Otherwise, everything just blurs.'

This module explores how structure—through meaningful rituals—can be a spark of healing, identity, and control.

Reflection Prompts

- What rituals do I already have in my life?
- Which routines give me comfort, predictability, or calm?
- Have I ever felt unsafe or lost when structure disappeared?
- What rituals connect me to my culture, family, or sense of self?
- Are there new rituals I want to create to support my well-being?

Spark Journal

Reflect on a daily or weekly ritual that gives you a sense of control, peace, or identity. Why does it matter to you?

_____

_____

_____

_____

_____

_____

_____

Try This: Build a Ritual Anchor

Choose one small ritual to do every day at the same time—lighting a candle, reciting a mantra, brewing tea, or taking a mindful breath. Let this anchor your day with consistency and meaning.

Clinician Insight

Rituals often reflect attempts to restore order or agency in lives disrupted by illness. Inquire about both comforting and compulsive rituals. Distinguish between adaptive routines and disabling rigidity. Ask: 'What daily rhythms help you feel grounded?' or 'Do you have any practices that help you feel more like yourself?' Structure can be therapeutic.

Module 9

Nature and Grounding: The Spark of Belonging, Stillness, and Earth Connection

Nature offers us something profound—a sense of grounding, rhythm, and perspective. For individuals living with serious mental illness, connection to the natural world can reduce stress, ease isolation, and offer moments of calm when everything else feels overwhelming.

One patient once said to me, 'When I'm outside, the voices quiet down. The trees don't judge me.' Nature doesn't require performance. It simply welcomes presence.

This module honors the spark of nature—not just wilderness, but also sunlight, fresh air, gardens, rain, and sky. These simple elements can restore a sense of rootedness and dignity.

Reflection Prompts

- When was the last time I felt peace outdoors?
- Are there natural places I return to for comfort or reflection?
- What textures, sounds, or sights in nature calm my nervous system?
- Have I ever had a healing experience in nature?
- How do I bring elements of nature into my daily space or routine?

Spark Journal

Describe a memory of being in nature that brought you peace or insight. What did your body feel like? What emotions came up?

_____

_____

_____

_____

_____

_____

_____

Try This: Grounding with the Earth

Step outside for five minutes. Focus on one natural object—a leaf, a stone, a patch of dirt. Hold it or sit near it. Breathe slowly. Let yourself remember: you are part of this world. Let the earth hold you.

Clinician Insight

Time in nature is linked to reduced anxiety, lower cortisol levels, and increased positive affect. For clients with severe mental illness, nature can offer non-verbal healing. Even a walk around the block, tending a plant, or looking out a window can foster regulation. Incorporate grounding techniques like '5-4-3-2-1 senses' in outdoor spaces when possible.

Module 10

Humor and Playfulness: The Spark of Lightness, Resilience, and Connection

We often think of healing as serious work—and it is. But sometimes, what keeps us going is a moment of absurdity, a shared laugh, or the ability to make light of our pain just enough to survive it. Humor doesn't erase suffering, but it creates space. It says: even here, even now, there's still room to breathe.

I remember a patient who brought rubber chickens to group therapy. When someone asked why, he replied, 'Because sometimes depression needs a punchline.' That moment lifted the whole room.

This module honors humor as a spark—not to dismiss pain, but to move through it. It's about reconnecting with joy, mischief, silliness, and the delight of being human.

Reflection Prompts

- What makes me laugh, even on hard days?
- When was the last time I felt playful, goofy, or free?
- Do I use humor to cope, connect, or deflect?
- Are there people in my life who help me laugh at myself kindly?
- What stories or jokes have helped me survive difficult experiences?

Spark Journal

Write about a time when laughter helped you get through something hard. Who were you with? How did it feel in your body?

_____

_____

_____

_____

_____

_____

_____

Try This: Find a Moment of Play

Watch a funny video, doodle a cartoon, dance badly to a song, or tell a ridiculous joke. Let yourself feel light—even for a few moments. Notice how it changes your energy.

Clinician Insight

Humor can signal resilience and cognitive flexibility. For patients, it can reduce stigma, build rapport, and enhance group dynamics. Play-based interventions, especially with youth or those with trauma, can support emotional expression and healing. Validate laughter as strength, not avoidance. Ask: 'What helps you laugh, even on the worst days?'

Module 11

Touch and Sensation: The Spark of Connection, Grounding, and Comfort

Touch is one of the first senses we develop—and often one of the most misunderstood. For people living with serious mental illness, touch can be healing or painful, comforting or triggering. Sensory experiences—warm blankets, firm handshakes, hugs, or textured fabrics—can all hold meaning. They remind the body that it is here. That it is real.

One patient told me, 'I wear a heavy scarf in summer, not for fashion, but because it's the only thing that keeps me from floating away.' This isn't metaphor. It's regulation.

This module explores how touch and sensation—through texture, weight, pressure, temperature, or movement—can anchor, soothe, and reconnect us.

Reflection Prompts

- How do I experience physical touch—with others or myself?
- Are there textures or sensations that bring me comfort?
- Do certain types of touch make me anxious or grounded?
- How do I regulate my emotions through physical sensations?
- What role has touch played in my healing or trauma journey?

Spark Journal

Describe a time when physical touch—yours or someone else's—helped you feel safe or connected. What was that moment like?

_____

_____

_____

_____

_____

_____

_____

_____

Try This: Sensory Scan

Find three textures you enjoy—a soft fabric, a smooth stone, warm water. Run your fingers across them slowly. Take note of your breathing. This is a sensory check-in. Let the body speak.

Clinician Insight

Touch can be deeply therapeutic—and deeply fraught. Trauma, neglect, or institutionalization often shape a patient's relationship with physical sensation. Somatic therapies, weighted blankets, and sensory kits may help. Inquire gently: 'What kinds of touch or sensations help you feel more in control—or more yourself?'

Module 12

Storytelling and Meaning-Making: The Spark of Narrative, Voice, and Self-Understanding

We live by stories. The ones we tell about ourselves. The ones others tell about us. The ones we're still trying to rewrite.

For people with serious mental illness, storytelling becomes more than expression—it becomes survival. It's a way to claim identity in the face of stigma, to say, 'I am more than my diagnosis.'

One patient shared, 'Every time I tell my story, it changes a little. Not because I'm lying—but because I'm healing.'

This module explores how narrative—through words, images, music, or memory—can shape meaning, dignity, and hope. Everyone has a story. The work is helping people feel safe enough to tell it.

Reflection Prompts

- What stories about myself have I internalized from others?
- Which parts of my story do I keep hidden, and why?
- What moments in my life shaped how I see myself?
- Have I ever felt transformed by telling or hearing a story?
- What kind of story do I want to tell moving forward?

Spark Journal

Write a brief version of your story—not your symptoms, but your soul. What do you want others to understand about you?

_____

_____

_____

_____

_____

_____

_____

Try This: Rewrite One Chapter

Think of a difficult chapter in your life. Now imagine retelling it with compassion—not as failure, but as survival. Use your own words, your own voice. You are the narrator.

Clinician Insight

Narrative therapy invites patients to explore meaning beyond pathology. Reframing language (e.g., from 'I'm broken' to 'I've endured') is powerful. Storytelling allows trauma integration, identity formation, and connection. Offer prompts like: 'If your story had a title, what would it be?' or 'What chapter are you in now?'

Module 13

Hope and Possibility: The Spark of Future, Faith, and Inner Light

Hope is not naive. It's radical. It insists that even in the depths of despair, some part of us still believes in tomorrow.

For people with serious mental illness, hope is not a cliché—it's a clinical necessity. Without it, there is no recovery, only maintenance. And yet, too often, systems extinguish it. They focus on compliance, not dreams. On stability, not possibility.

One patient told me, 'I just want someone to believe I'm not done yet.' That's what this module is about.

Hope doesn't always come with fireworks. Sometimes it shows up as a whisper, a single step, a gentle nudge toward the light.

Reflection Prompts

- What keeps me going, even when things are hard?
- Have I ever felt hopeless—and what helped shift that feeling?
- Who in my life holds hope for me when I can't?
- What dreams or goals do I still carry, however quietly?
- What does hope look like for me now—not as fantasy, but as possibility?

Spark Journal

Write a letter to your future self—reminding them what you've already survived and why you're still here.

_____
_____
_____
_____
_____
_____
_____

Try This: Name the Next Step

Think of one small thing you can do this week that moves you toward something you want. Not a giant leap—just a spark of movement. Write it down. Tell someone. Hope is action.

Clinician Insight

Hope is associated with better treatment adherence, improved resilience, and lower suicidality. Micro-goal setting, narrative reframing, and peer models of recovery can nurture it. Ask: 'What's something you're still hoping for?' or 'Can we imagine the next chapter together?' Even naming hope is an intervention.

Module 14

Freedom and Autonomy: The Spark of Choice, Agency, and Dignity

Freedom is more than civil rights—it's deeply personal. For people with serious mental illness, it often feels like the first thing taken away.

Whether it's hospitalization, forced medication, conservatorship, or stigma, many individuals experience a world that limits their autonomy.

And yet—within those constraints, people still seek ways to choose: what to wear, what music to play, when to rest, who to trust.

I remember a patient who refused all treatment—until a nurse said, 'We won't force anything. But we will walk with you.' That changed everything.

This module honors the human need to decide one's own path, even when that path looks different than what others expect.

Reflection Prompts

- When do I feel most in control of my own life?
- What decisions am I allowed to make—and which ones feel out of reach?
- Have I ever felt like my freedom was taken from me?
- What helps me reclaim my sense of agency?
- How do I want to define dignity for myself?

Spark Journal

Describe a time when you made a choice—big or small—that reminded you of your power. What did it feel like?

_____

_____

_____

_____

_____

_____

_____

Try This: Make One Liberating Choice

Today, choose something entirely for you. It might be a boundary, an outfit, a walk, a song. Let this act remind you that your life is your own.

Clinician Insight

Autonomy is a core component of recovery-oriented care. Even when choices are limited, supporting decision-making builds trust and empowerment. Offer collaborative care plans, shared decision tools, and space for disagreement. Ask: 'What's something you'd like to decide for yourself today?' Respecting choice—even in small ways—restores dignity.

Module 15
SPARK ASSESSMENT TOOL

Spark Self-Assessment Tool (General)

For individuals, families, and peers to explore which core human drives or sparks are most present, missing, or dormant in life.

Instructions:
1. Read each statement for every spark.
2. Rate how true it feels right now using the 0–4 scale:
   - 0 = Not at all true for me
   - 1 = A little bit true
   - 2 = Somewhat true
   - 3 = Mostly true
   - 4 = Very true
3. Add up your points for each spark to get a Total Score out of 16.
4. Use the scoring guide to interpret your results.

Scoring Guide

Per Spark (0–16 points):
- 0–4 → Spark is largely absent; might need intentional support or exploration.
- 5–8 → Spark is emerging; some engagement but not yet consistent or fulfilling.
- 9–12 → Spark is active; meaningful presence with room for growth.
- 13–16 → Spark is strong; well-integrated and a source of energy in life.

Overall Spark Profile:
- High total score across most sparks → Well-rounded engagement with multiple life-affirming drives.
- High variation between sparks → Possible areas of neglect, imbalance, or untapped potential.
- Multiple low scores → May indicate reduced quality of life, isolation, or lack of access to fulfilling activities.

Sex and Intimacy

1. I currently feel connected to this spark.
2. This area brings me joy, meaning, or energy.
3. I have ways to access or engage with this spark regularly.
4. I would like to explore or strengthen this spark more.

Total Score: _____ / 16

Notes:
_____
_____

Money and Security

1. I currently feel connected to this spark.
2. This area brings me joy, meaning, or energy.
3. I have ways to access or engage with this spark regularly.
4. I would like to explore or strengthen this spark more.

Total Score: _____ / 16

Notes:
_____
_____

Food and Nourishment

1. I currently feel connected to this spark.
2. This area brings me joy, meaning, or energy.
3. I have ways to access or engage with this spark regularly.
4. I would like to explore or strengthen this spark more.

Total Score: _____ / 16

Notes:
_____
_____

Music and Resonance

1. I currently feel connected to this spark.
2. This area brings me joy, meaning, or energy.
3. I have ways to access or engage with this spark regularly.
4. I would like to explore or strengthen this spark more.

Total Score: _____ / 16

Notes:
_____
_____

Spirituality and Meaning

1. I currently feel connected to this spark.
2. This area brings me joy, meaning, or energy.
3. I have ways to access or engage with this spark regularly.
4. I would like to explore or strengthen this spark more.

Total Score: _____ / 16

Notes:
_____
_____

Creativity and Expression

1. I currently feel connected to this spark.
2. This area brings me joy, meaning, or energy.
3. I have ways to access or engage with this spark regularly.
4. I would like to explore or strengthen this spark more.

Total Score: _____ / 16

Notes:
_____
_____

Movement and Embodiment

1. I currently feel connected to this spark.
2. This area brings me joy, meaning, or energy.
3. I have ways to access or engage with this spark regularly.
4. I would like to explore or strengthen this spark more.

Total Score: _____ / 16

Notes:
_____
_____

Rituals and Structure

1. I currently feel connected to this spark.
2. This area brings me joy, meaning, or energy.
3. I have ways to access or engage with this spark regularly.
4. I would like to explore or strengthen this spark more.

Total Score: _____ / 16

Notes:
_____
_____

Nature and Grounding

1. I currently feel connected to this spark.
2. This area brings me joy, meaning, or energy.
3. I have ways to access or engage with this spark regularly.
4. I would like to explore or strengthen this spark more.

Total Score: _____ / 16

Notes:
_____
_____

Humor and Playfulness

1. I currently feel connected to this spark.
2. This area brings me joy, meaning, or energy.
3. I have ways to access or engage with this spark regularly.
4. I would like to explore or strengthen this spark more.

Total Score: _____ / 16

Notes:
_____
_____

Touch and Sensation

1. I currently feel connected to this spark.
2. This area brings me joy, meaning, or energy.
3. I have ways to access or engage with this spark regularly.
4. I would like to explore or strengthen this spark more.

Total Score: _____ / 16

Notes:
_____
_____

Storytelling and Meaning-Making

1. I currently feel connected to this spark.
2. This area brings me joy, meaning, or energy.
3. I have ways to access or engage with this spark regularly.
4. I would like to explore or strengthen this spark more.

Total Score: _____ / 16

Notes:
_____
_____

Hope and Possibility

1. I currently feel connected to this spark.
2. This area brings me joy, meaning, or energy.
3. I have ways to access or engage with this spark regularly.
4. I would like to explore or strengthen this spark more.

Total Score: _____ / 16

Notes:
_____
_____

Freedom and Autonomy

1. I currently feel connected to this spark.
2. This area brings me joy, meaning, or energy.
3. I have ways to access or engage with this spark regularly.
4. I would like to explore or strengthen this spark more.

Total Score: _____ / 16

Notes:
_____
_____

Clinician Sparks Assessment Tool

Purpose:

Helps clinicians identify which sparks are present, absent, misunderstood, or stigmatized and where to intervene for recovery-oriented growth.

How to Use:
- Can be used in intake, treatment planning, or progress reviews.
- Check relevant boxes and fill in Opportunities and Clinical Actions.

Sex and Intimacy

☐ Spark appears present
☐ Spark appears limited or absent
☐ Spark is misunderstood, stigmatized, or pathologized

Opportunities to strengthen or reframe this spark:

_____

_____

Clinical action or goal:

_____

_____

Money and Security

☐ Spark appears present
☐ Spark appears limited or absent
☐ Spark is misunderstood, stigmatized, or pathologized

Opportunities to strengthen or reframe this spark:

_____

_____

Clinical action or goal:

_____

_____

Food and Nourishment

☐ Spark appears present
☐ Spark appears limited or absent
☐ Spark is misunderstood, stigmatized, or pathologized

Opportunities to strengthen or reframe this spark:

_____
_____

Clinical action or goal:

_____
_____

Music and Resonance

☐ Spark appears present
☐ Spark appears limited or absent
☐ Spark is misunderstood, stigmatized, or pathologized

Opportunities to strengthen or reframe this spark:

_____
_____

Clinical action or goal:

_____
_____

Spirituality and Meaning

☐ Spark appears present
☐ Spark appears limited or absent
☐ Spark is misunderstood, stigmatized, or pathologized

Opportunities to strengthen or reframe this spark:

_____
_____

Clinical action or goal:

_____
_____

Creativity and Expression

☐ Spark appears present
☐ Spark appears limited or absent
☐ Spark is misunderstood, stigmatized, or pathologized

Opportunities to strengthen or reframe this spark:

_____
_____

Clinical action or goal:

_____
_____

Movement and Embodiment

☐ Spark appears present
☐ Spark appears limited or absent
☐ Spark is misunderstood, stigmatized, or pathologized

Opportunities to strengthen or reframe this spark:

_____
_____

Clinical action or goal:

_____
_____

Rituals and Structure

☐ Spark appears present
☐ Spark appears limited or absent
☐ Spark is misunderstood, stigmatized, or pathologized

Opportunities to strengthen or reframe this spark:

_____
_____

Clinical action or goal:

_____
_____

Nature and Grounding

☐ Spark appears present
☐ Spark appears limited or absent
☐ Spark is misunderstood, stigmatized, or pathologized

Opportunities to strengthen or reframe this spark:
_____
_____

Clinical action or goal:
_____
_____

Humor and Playfulness

☐ Spark appears present
☐ Spark appears limited or absent
☐ Spark is misunderstood, stigmatized, or pathologized

Opportunities to strengthen or reframe this spark:
_____
_____

Clinical action or goal:
_____
_____

Touch and Sensation

☐ Spark appears present
☐ Spark appears limited or absent
☐ Spark is misunderstood, stigmatized, or pathologized

Opportunities to strengthen or reframe this spark:
_____
_____

Clinical action or goal:
_____
_____

Storytelling and Meaning-Making

☐ Spark appears present
☐ Spark appears limited or absent
☐ Spark is misunderstood, stigmatized, or pathologized

Opportunities to strengthen or reframe this spark:

_____

_____

Clinical action or goal:

_____

_____

Hope and Possibility

☐ Spark appears present
☐ Spark appears limited or absent
☐ Spark is misunderstood, stigmatized, or pathologized

Opportunities to strengthen or reframe this spark:

_____

_____

Clinical action or goal:

_____

Freedom and Autonomy

☐ Spark appears present
☐ Spark appears limited or absent
☐ Spark is misunderstood, stigmatized, or pathologized

Opportunities to strengthen or reframe this spark:

_____

_____

Clinical action or goal:

_____

Spark Profile Summary Sheet

Use this sheet to record your total score for each spark after completing the self-assessment. This gives you a quick view of your strongest and weakest areas.

Spark	Total Score (0–16)	Quick Notes / Observations
Sex and Intimacy	_____	
Money and Security	_____	
Food and Nourishment	_____	
Music and Resonance	_____	
Spirituality and Meaning	_____	
Creativity and Expression	_____	
Movement and Embodiment	_____	
Rituals and Structure	_____	
Nature and Grounding	_____	
Humor and Playfulness	_____	
Touch and Sensation	_____	
Storytelling and Meaning-Making	_____	
Hope and Possibility	_____	
Freedom and Autonomy	_____	
TOTAL SCORE (All Sparks Combined)	_____ / 224	

Reflection & Journaling: Sex and Intimacy

What does this spark mean to you personally?

Have you seen it show up in your own recovery or in others?

Where is this spark blocked or missing in your life?

What small step could help reignite this spark?

Notes:

_____
_____
_____
_____
_____
_____
_____
_____
_____
_____

Patient Vignette Example – Sex and Intimacy

When I first reconnected physically with my partner after months apart, I realized intimacy wasn't just physical, it was a bridge back to trust.

Clinical Insight

Clinicians can explore how this spark intersects with symptoms, trauma history, medication side effects, or systemic barriers. Use motivational interviewing to ask: 'When was the last time this brought you joy?' or 'What would help you reconnect with this part of yourself?'

Summary Worksheet

Spark Status: ☐ Present ☐ Missing ☐ Repressed

My Next Action Step: _____

Support Needed: _____

Reflection Word or Image: _____

Reflection & Journaling: Money and Security

What does this spark mean to you personally?

Have you seen it show up in your own recovery or in others?

Where is this spark blocked or missing in your life?

What small step could help reignite this spark?

Notes:
_____
_____
_____
_____
_____
_____
_____
_____
_____
_____

Patient Vignette Example – Money and Security

When I finally saved enough for my own apartment, I felt a sense of security I hadn't experienced since before my diagnosis.

Clinical Insight

Clinicians can explore how this spark intersects with symptoms, trauma history, medication side effects, or systemic barriers. Use motivational interviewing to ask: 'When was the last time this brought you joy?' or 'What would help you reconnect with this part of yourself?'

Summary Worksheet

Spark Status: ☐ Present ☐ Missing ☐ Repressed

My Next Action Step: _____

Support Needed: _____

Reflection Word or Image: _____

Reflection & Journaling: Food and Nourishment

What does this spark mean to you personally?

Have you seen it show up in your own recovery or in others?

Where is this spark blocked or missing in your life?

What small step could help reignite this spark?

Notes:

_____
_____
_____
_____
_____
_____
_____
_____
_____
_____

Patient Vignette Example – Food and Nourishment

When I started cooking my grandmother's recipes again, I felt nourished in both body and memory.

Clinical Insight

Clinicians can explore how this spark intersects with symptoms, trauma history, medication side effects, or systemic barriers. Use motivational interviewing to ask: 'When was the last time this brought you joy?' or 'What would help you reconnect with this part of yourself?'

Summary Worksheet

Spark Status: ☐ Present ☐ Missing ☐ Repressed

My Next Action Step: _____

Support Needed: _____

Reflection Word or Image: _____

Reflection & Journaling: Music and Resonance

What does this spark mean to you personally?

Have you seen it show up in your own recovery or in others?

Where is this spark blocked or missing in your life?

What small step could help reignite this spark?

Notes:
_____
_____
_____
_____
_____
_____
_____
_____
_____
_____

Patient Vignette Example – Music and Resonance

When I picked up my guitar after years of silence, each chord reminded me I was still here, still creating.

Clinical Insight

Clinicians can explore how this spark intersects with symptoms, trauma history, medication side effects, or systemic barriers. Use motivational interviewing to ask: 'When was the last time this brought you joy?' or 'What would help you reconnect with this part of yourself?'

Summary Worksheet

Spark Status: ☐ Present ☐ Missing ☐ Repressed

My Next Action Step: _____

Support Needed: _____

Reflection Word or Image: _____

Reflection & Journaling: Spirituality and Meaning

What does this spark mean to you personally?

Have you seen it show up in your own recovery or in others?

Where is this spark blocked or missing in your life?

What small step could help reignite this spark?

Notes:

_____
_____
_____
_____
_____
_____
_____
_____
_____
_____

Patient Vignette Example – Spirituality and Meaning

When I returned to my faith community, the shared prayers felt like a lifeline pulling me toward hope.

Clinical Insight

Clinicians can explore how this spark intersects with symptoms, trauma history, medication side effects, or systemic barriers. Use motivational interviewing to ask: 'When was the last time this brought you joy?' or 'What would help you reconnect with this part of yourself?'

Summary Worksheet

Spark Status: ☐ Present ☐ Missing ☐ Repressed

My Next Action Step: _____

Support Needed: _____

Reflection Word or Image: _____

Reflection & Journaling: Creativity and Expression

What does this spark mean to you personally?

Have you seen it show up in your own recovery or in others?

Where is this spark blocked or missing in your life?

What small step could help reignite this spark?

Notes:
_____
_____
_____
_____
_____
_____
_____
_____
_____
_____

Patient Vignette Example – Creativity and Expression

When I painted my first canvas after treatment, I saw my healing reflected in the colors.

Clinical Insight

Clinicians can explore how this spark intersects with symptoms, trauma history, medication side effects, or systemic barriers. Use motivational interviewing to ask: 'When was the last time this brought you joy?' or 'What would help you reconnect with this part of yourself?'

Summary Worksheet

Spark Status: ☐ Present ☐ Missing ☐ Repressed

My Next Action Step: _____

Support Needed: _____

Reflection Word or Image: _____

Reflection & Journaling: Movement and Embodiment

What does this spark mean to you personally?

Have you seen it show up in your own recovery or in others?

Where is this spark blocked or missing in your life?

What small step could help reignite this spark?

Notes:
_____
_____
_____
_____
_____
_____
_____
_____
_____
_____

Patient Vignette Example – Movement and Embodiment

When I began daily morning walks, I felt my body and mind rejoin in quiet conversation.

Clinical Insight

Clinicians can explore how this spark intersects with symptoms, trauma history, medication side effects, or systemic barriers. Use motivational interviewing to ask: 'When was the last time this brought you joy?' or 'What would help you reconnect with this part of yourself?'

Summary Worksheet

Spark Status: ☐ Present ☐ Missing ☐ Repressed

My Next Action Step: _____

Support Needed: _____

Reflection Word or Image: _____

Reflection & Journaling: Rituals and Structure

What does this spark mean to you personally?

Have you seen it show up in your own recovery or in others?

Where is this spark blocked or missing in your life?

What small step could help reignite this spark?

Notes:
_____
_____
_____
_____
_____
_____
_____
_____
_____
_____
_____

Patient Vignette Example – Rituals and Structure

When I lit a candle every night before bed, my days began and ended with a comforting rhythm.

Clinical Insight

Clinicians can explore how this spark intersects with symptoms, trauma history, medication side effects, or systemic barriers. Use motivational interviewing to ask: 'When was the last time this brought you joy?' or 'What would help you reconnect with this part of yourself?'

Summary Worksheet

Spark Status: ☐ Present ☐ Missing ☐ Repressed

My Next Action Step: _____

Support Needed: _____

Reflection Word or Image: _____

Reflection & Journaling: Nature and Grounding

What does this spark mean to you personally?

Have you seen it show up in your own recovery or in others?

Where is this spark blocked or missing in your life?

What small step could help reignite this spark?

Notes:

_____
_____
_____
_____
_____
_____
_____
_____
_____
_____

Patient Vignette Example – Nature and Grounding

When I sat under the oak tree in my yard, the steady rustle of leaves anchored me in the present.

Clinical Insight

Clinicians can explore how this spark intersects with symptoms, trauma history, medication side effects, or systemic barriers. Use motivational interviewing to ask: 'When was the last time this brought you joy?' or 'What would help you reconnect with this part of yourself?'

Summary Worksheet

Spark Status: ☐ Present ☐ Missing ☐ Repressed

My Next Action Step: _____

Support Needed: _____

Reflection Word or Image: _____

Reflection & Journaling: Humor and Playfulness

What does this spark mean to you personally?

Have you seen it show up in your own recovery or in others?

Where is this spark blocked or missing in your life?

What small step could help reignite this spark?

Notes:
_____
_____
_____
_____
_____
_____
_____
_____
_____
_____

Patient Vignette Example – Humor and Playfulness

When I started telling silly jokes at group therapy, the laughter reminded us we were more than our diagnoses.

Clinical Insight

Clinicians can explore how this spark intersects with symptoms, trauma history, medication side effects, or systemic barriers. Use motivational interviewing to ask: 'When was the last time this brought you joy?' or 'What would help you reconnect with this part of yourself?'

Summary Worksheet

Spark Status: ☐ Present ☐ Missing ☐ Repressed

My Next Action Step: _____

Support Needed: _____

Reflection Word or Image: _____

Reflection & Journaling: Touch and Sensation

What does this spark mean to you personally?

Have you seen it show up in your own recovery or in others?

Where is this spark blocked or missing in your life?

What small step could help reignite this spark?

Notes:

_____
_____
_____
_____
_____
_____
_____
_____
_____
_____

Patient Vignette Example – Touch and Sensation

When my niece hugged me tightly, I felt the warmth ripple through my whole being.

Clinical Insight

Clinicians can explore how this spark intersects with symptoms, trauma history, medication side effects, or systemic barriers. Use motivational interviewing to ask: 'When was the last time this brought you joy?' or 'What would help you reconnect with this part of yourself?'

Summary Worksheet

Spark Status: ☐ Present ☐ Missing ☐ Repressed

My Next Action Step: _____

Support Needed: _____

Reflection Word or Image: _____

Reflection & Journaling: Storytelling and Meaning-Making

What does this spark mean to you personally?

Have you seen it show up in your own recovery or in others?

Where is this spark blocked or missing in your life?

What small step could help reignite this spark?

Notes:
_____
_____
_____
_____
_____
_____
_____
_____
_____
_____

Patient Vignette Example – Storytelling and Meaning-Making

When I shared my recovery story at a support group, I realized my words could light the way for others.

Clinical Insight

Clinicians can explore how this spark intersects with symptoms, trauma history, medication side effects, or systemic barriers. Use motivational interviewing to ask: 'When was the last time this brought you joy?' or 'What would help you reconnect with this part of yourself?'

Summary Worksheet

Spark Status: ☐ Present ☐ Missing ☐ Repressed

My Next Action Step: _____

Support Needed: _____

Reflection Word or Image: _____

Reflection & Journaling: Hope and Possibility

What does this spark mean to you personally?

Have you seen it show up in your own recovery or in others?

Where is this spark blocked or missing in your life?

What small step could help reignite this spark?

Notes:

_____

_____

_____

_____

_____

_____

_____

_____

_____

_____

Patient Vignette Example – Hope and Possibility

When I planted seeds in my garden, I saw a vision of tomorrow taking root.

Clinical Insight

Clinicians can explore how this spark intersects with symptoms, trauma history, medication side effects, or systemic barriers. Use motivational interviewing to ask: 'When was the last time this brought you joy?' or 'What would help you reconnect with this part of yourself?'

Summary Worksheet

Spark Status: ☐ Present ☐ Missing ☐ Repressed

My Next Action Step: _____

Support Needed: _____

Reflection Word or Image: _____

Reflection & Journaling: Freedom and Autonomy

What does this spark mean to you personally?

Have you seen it show up in your own recovery or in others?

Where is this spark blocked or missing in your life?

What small step could help reignite this spark?

Notes:
_____
_____
_____
_____
_____
_____
_____
_____
_____
_____

Patient Vignette Example – Freedom and Autonomy

When I got my driver's license back, the open road felt like a promise fulfilled.

Clinical Insight

Clinicians can explore how this spark intersects with symptoms, trauma history, medication side effects, or systemic barriers. Use motivational interviewing to ask: 'When was the last time this brought you joy?' or 'What would help you reconnect with this part of yourself?'

Summary Worksheet

Spark Status: ☐ Present ☐ Missing ☐ Repressed

My Next Action Step: _____

Support Needed: _____

Reflection Word or Image: _____

Final Notes & Reflections

"Even the darkest night will end and the sun will rise."
— Victor Hugo

"Recovery is not a race. You don't have to feel guilty if it takes you longer than you thought it would."

"There is a crack in everything, that's how the light gets in."
— Leonard Cohen

"Hope is being able to see that there is light despite all of the darkness." — Desmond Tutu

"The human spirit is stronger than anything that can happen to it." — C.C. Scott

"Sometimes music is the only medicine the heart and soul need."

"Creativity takes courage."
— Henri Matisse

> *"Movement is a medicine for creating change in a person's physical, emotional, and mental states."*
> — Carol Welch

"Rituals are the formulas by which harmony is restored."
— Terry Tempest Williams

> *"Nature is not a place to visit. It is home."*
> — Gary Snyder

> **"*Laughter is the shortest distance between two people.*"**
> — Victor Borge

"Touch comes before sight, before speech. It is the first language and the last." — Margaret Atwood

"The most powerful person in the world is the storyteller."
— Steve Jobs

> *"Hope is the pillar that holds up the world."*
> — Pliny the Elder

The Spark Wheel

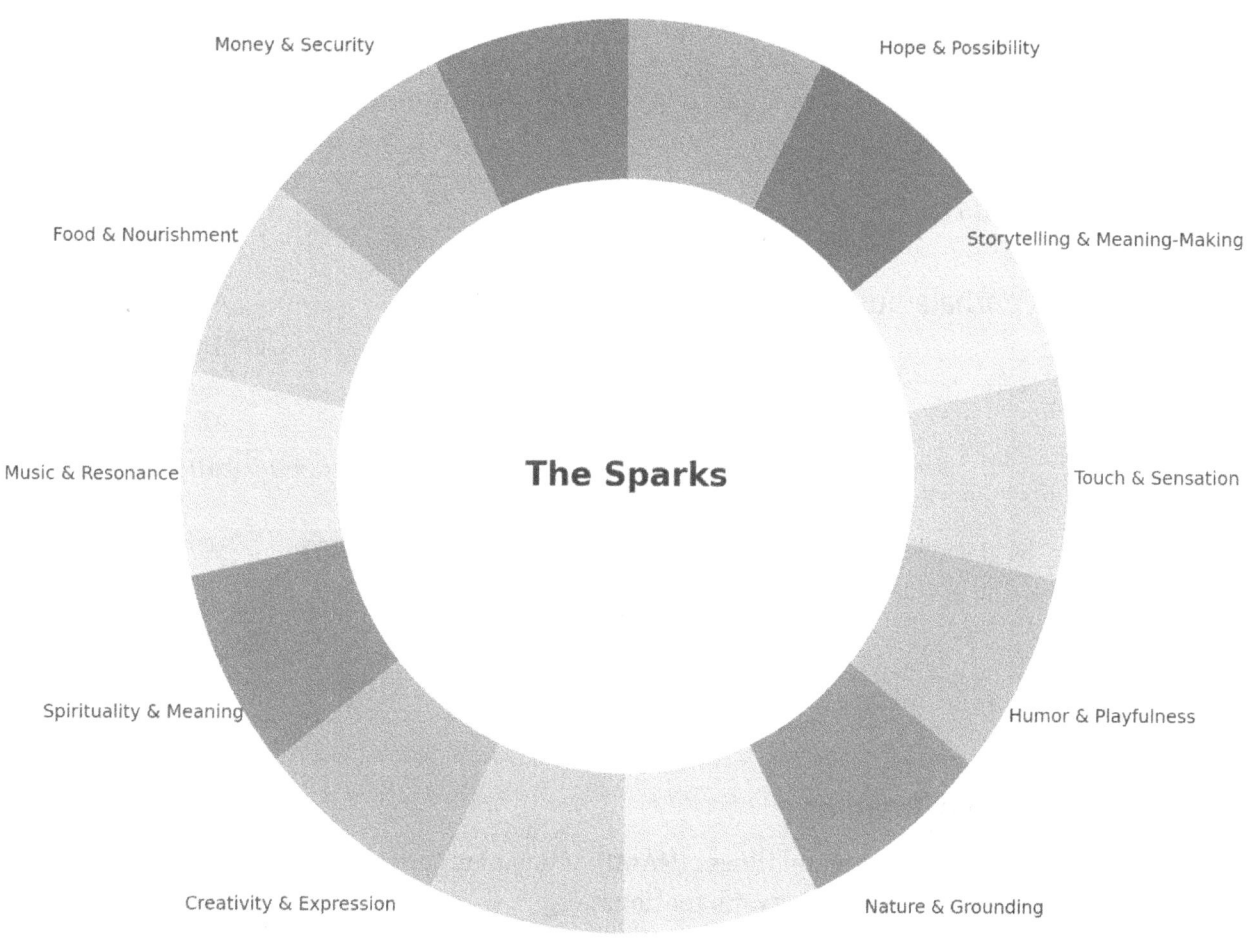

Diagram: Brain Regions Associated with Sparks

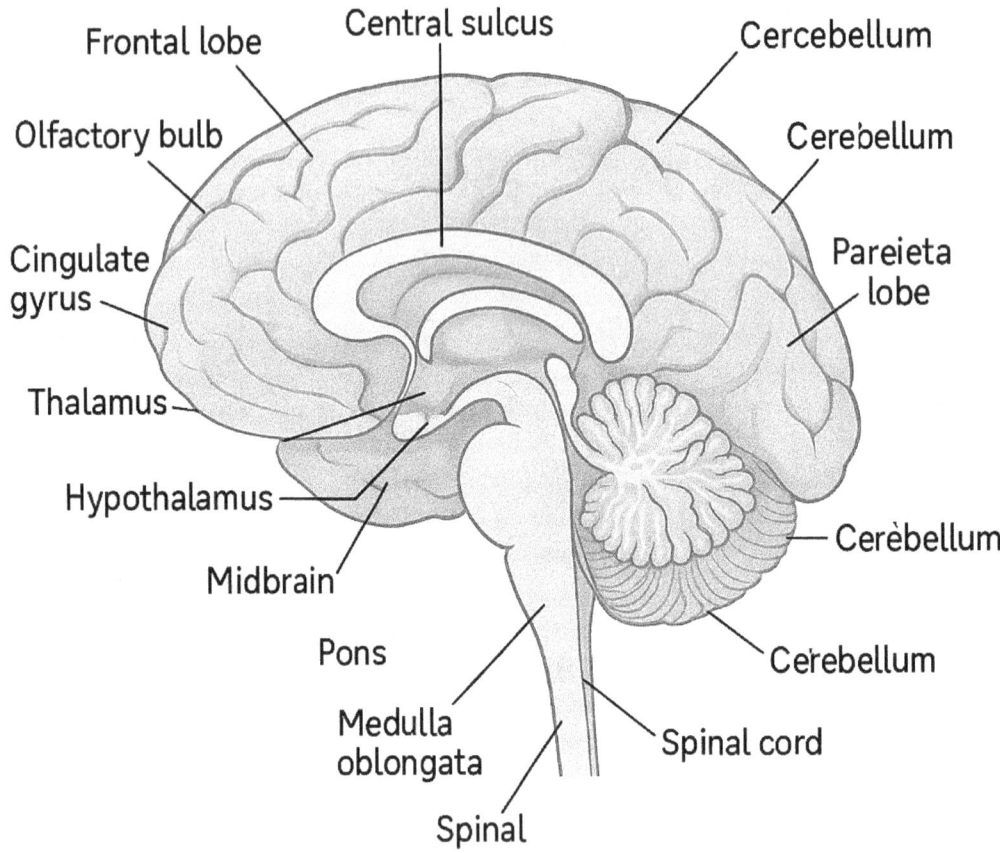

Resources & Further Reading

- National Alliance on Mental Illness (NAMI): www.nami.org
- Mental Health America: www.mhanational.org
- Crisis Text Line: Text HOME to 741741
- SAMHSA Treatment Locator: findtreatment.gov
- The Sparks That Endure by Clovis Raymond, MD (Main Book)
- Psychology Today Therapy Directory: www.psychologytoday.com

Personal Notes

More Notes

Module 16

Conclusion and Reflection: Carrying the Spark Forward

If you've made it this far, thank you. Whether you joined this journey as a clinician, a caregiver, a peer, or someone seeking healing, I hope this workbook reminded you of something essential:

Even when minds are chaotic, even when systems fail, even when words are lost—something meaningful still burns inside.

The sparks we explored—sex, money, food, music, faith, creativity, movement, rituals, nature, humor, touch, storytelling, hope, and freedom—aren't extras. They are the core of what it means to be human.

This work was never just academic. It was personal. I found myself awake at 4:30 AM, still writing. My daughters shook me awake a couple hours later. I was exhausted—and alive. That's the paradox of a spark. It burns, but it also fuels.

Now it's your turn. What will you do with what you've discovered? Will you see someone differently? Reconnect with your own spark? Shift how you ask questions or hold space?

Wherever you go from here, I hope you remember:

The spark remains. Always. Even in darkness.

Clovis Raymond, MD

Final Reflection Prompts

- Which spark resonated most deeply with me—and why?
- How have my views on mental illness and recovery shifted?
- What practices or habits do I want to carry forward?
- How can I support others in reconnecting with their sparks?
- What do I want to remember when things feel dark again?

Spark Journal

What does it mean to you to be fully alive? Describe your vision of a life with your spark fully ignited.

_____
_____
_____
_____
_____
_____
_____

Try This: Spark Commitment

Write down one commitment to yourself—a promise to nurture one spark in your life. Sign it, date it, and place it somewhere you'll see.

Today, I commit to _____

Date: _____ Signature: _____

References

American Psychiatric Association. (2013). *Diagnostic and statistical manual of mental disorders* (5th ed.). American Psychiatric Publishing.

Bassuk, E. L., Dawson, R., Huntington, N., et al. (2006). Characteristics and needs of victims of domestic violence with psychiatric disabilities. *Psychiatric Services*, 57(5), 620–626.

Deci, E. L., & Ryan, R. M. (2000). The 'what' and 'why' of goal pursuits: Human needs and the self-determination of behavior. *Psychological Inquiry*, 11(4), 227–268.

Fosha, D. (2000). *The transforming power of affect: A model for accelerated change.* Basic Books.

Herman, J. L. (1992). *Trauma and recovery: The aftermath of violence—from domestic abuse to political terror.* Basic Books.

Koenig, H. G. (2009). *Religion and mental health: Research and clinical applications.* Academic Press.

LeDoux, J. (2002). *Synaptic self: How our brains become who we are.* Penguin Books.

Masten, A. S. (2001). Ordinary magic: Resilience processes in development. *American Psychologist*, 56(3), 227–238.

McGonigal, K. (2015). *The upside of stress: Why stress is good for you, and how to get good at it.* Avery.

Perry, B. D., & Szalavitz, M. (2006). *The boy who was raised as a dog: And other stories from a child psychiatrist's notebook.* Basic Books.

Siegel, D. J. (2012). *The developing mind: How relationships and the brain interact to shape who we are.* Guilford Press.

Van der Kolk, B. A. (2014). *The body keeps the score: Brain, mind, and body in the healing of trauma.* Viking.

Yalom, I. D. (2008). *Staring at the sun: Overcoming the terror of death.* Jossey-Bass.

Raymond, C. (2025). *The sparks that endure: Why our core human drives survive mental illness.* Clovis Raymond Group, LLC.

About the Author

Clovis Raymond, MD, is a **dual board-certified psychiatrist** in General Adult Psychiatry and Child & Adolescent Psychiatry. He serves as **Chief of Psychiatry at Rockland Psychiatric Center** in New York and **Assistant Clinical Professor of Psychiatry at Columbia University**, where he teaches trauma-informed and recovery-oriented care.

Dr. Raymond is the founder of **Clovis Raymond Group, LLC**, which develops **CME/CEU-accredited educational programs** that promote humane, person-centered psychiatry. With over two decades of experience treating individuals with schizophrenia, bipolar disorder, and related conditions, his work blends neuroscience, compassion, and cultural insight to illuminate what endures in the human spirit—even in illness.

The Sparks That Endure is his first major book.